All you need to know about Anal In a Quick Handbook

by

Vincent Ciofani

Real info from a real transsexual who practices the lifestyle daily.

Rather than have a big long book requiring a table of contents and a whole lot of unnecessary banter. This quick handbook will dive right into the ancient art of making one's anus double as a vagina.

Chapter 1

Proper anal lubricant

First things first would be to understand the best lubricant to have handy for anal sex. The best anal lube is plain old vegetable shortening, unflavored. Anything with flavor or scent can cause irritation of the inner anal membrane and unwanted constriction will result. That's why so many available KY and lube products are not necessarily the best to use for anal sex. If the anus becomes irritated inside, then there's less ability to relax and allow the penetration and the intercourse will be painful. Plus, due to the over-tightening of the irritated anus, the intercourse is less enjoyable for the penetrator.

Anything that will burn your butt should be avoided. You can have vegetable shortening ready in a container for use at your convenience. There should always be some at the ready in the bathroom where you defecate the most, and as an integral part of your portable sex kit. A proper amount of lubricant to apply would be to make sure that the anus is lubed up and that the penis (or penis substitute) is also lubricated. After some rigorous intercourse, the anus will start to lubricate itself.

Preparing for Anal Sex

Although the techniques you're about to learn may seem nasty upon presentation, there's nothing nastier than anal sex that was not prepared for. Plus, it can be uncomfortable because, the colon has a load in it, the lower anal cavity will barely be able to tolerate the intrusion. It will be less enjoyable, maybe even painful (in the bad way), and can be messy. However, one can reach a state of perpetual readiness for anal sex, with diet, technique, and practice. That begins with preparation prior to preparing.

Eating right is important. The goal is to have healthy feces that are not overly soft and runny. Beer and some foods contribute to an anal nastiness condition that can make preparation during defecation a tedious task. Eating more steak and salad and fiber helps to get this first stage set. Paying closer attention to what effects various foods have on your defecation process can afford huge advantages, later. You can learn to avoid things that tend to make you have nasty, unmanageable dukeys.

Doing The Two Finger Dig-out

On the toilet, after you defecate, clean your anus with toilet paper and then lubricate your middle finger with a small amount of your handy vegetable shortening. Reach down between your legs and lube your anus with the lubed finger. Once your anus is lubricated, insert your middle finger and move it all around inside your anus. Make sure to have toilet paper ready in your other hand to immediately clean off your finger and anus. Repeat this process a few times to remove the loose matter from the lower anal cavity. Clean off your anus and lubricate your finger between each insertion.

Once your middle finger is coming out with less dukey on it, repeat the process with two fingers. When you insert both fingers, move your fingers in a reaching motion alternating between the two (reach with one finger, then the other), as if you're trying to grab the inner walls of your anus just beyond the reach of your fingers.

[If you're a male, you'll feel a small ball that your fingers will pull against while doing this. That would be your prostate. Leave it in there.]

The desired result of this two fingered dig-out is to make the anal muscles force out any fecal matter that did not already come out. You may have to do this dig-out (and clean-up in-between) multiple times before getting everthing out. Keep doing this until your fingers come out clean, or with nothing on them except for vegetable shortening, and maybe some clear liquid.

You can acquire a state of perpetual preparedness that leaves your anus clean inside, odorless, and dripping wet with a clear liquid that resembles vaginal fluid. It all depends on your own level of commitment. The more anal sex you have, the more work you may have to exert to complete this process at times.

Your anus will now be ready for intercourse. Once you live the lifestyle of applying everything in this handbook, you may even be happily surprised with some involuntary anal squirting during unanticipated inner anal orgasms.

Chapter 2

When to enema:

Some erroneously believe that it's best to induce an enema prior to anal sex. But, if you have an enema and then have anal sex too closely afterward, it could be even more messy, as in really messy (and more nasty, too), than had you gone completely unprepared. If you insist on the enema prior to anal sex, then you should do so at least five to seven hours prior to having the intercourse, and the two fingered dig-out (immediately before sex) is still necessary for that confidence in cleanliness. If you squirt during intercourse, you want it to be clear, clean liquid. I should mention that one should try to be as clean as possible down there prior to administrating an enema for best results. So, the two fingered dig-out is a part of the process at the start and at the end of enemas, as well. Plus, for the after procedure I'll get into, later.

How To Enema

If you are going to use coffee for an enema, you should prepare your coffee and cool it with ice or cool water. You can leave the fluid warm if you prefer, but not hot. If you leave it too hot, you may damage your innards.

The open end stream adapter on the end of the hose is the smartest choice. Fill your enema bag and put the hose on it. Make sure the clamp is closed on the hose and leave the bag in the sink for now.

On the commode, use the two fingered dig-out method to make sure that there is no dukey to impede the deep penetration of the hose. Once your lower G.I. is clean, you can proceed to strategically hang your enema bag. You want it high enough to provide gravitational pull on the fluid. You'll find that you must compromise with the length of the hose sometimes. Holding the hose tip over the sink, tub, or toilet, open the clip to let a little of the fluid spray out and quickly close the clip (you don't want to lose too much fluid). This is to remove excess air from the hose. Make sure that the clip is at least 7 inches away from the insertion end of the hose to allow for deep penetration.

Now, get on your knees in front of the commode where you already have dark towels placed on the floor for you to crouch over. Slowly and carefully insert the end of the hose into your anus. With a slow inward and outward motion, work the hose deeper into your anus. The object is to get the hose deep without bending it inside of your butt. If you bend it, you'll splash fluid all over the floor and cause major discomfort when you open the clip. With some practice, you'll learn how to tell when you've bent the hose before making the ugly splash mess that you're bound to make at least once in your life.

With the hose deep into your anus, open the clip and bend down to the floor to assist gravity in pulling the fluid up into your intestines. You can arch your back and bounce a bit to help it along if preferred. You may have to pull the hose out a slight bit to get the flow started. You also may want to keep a hand on the hose so that it doesn't work its way out. The farther in you have it, the better the results. The desired depth will vary, anywhere between four inches and eight inches. Some people have better results with deeper penetration while others do not.

Your enema bag should be emptying. You should be able to see that it's getting flatter. Once you've taken as much of the fluid as you can, close the clip and slowly remove the hose from your anus. Set the enema bag in the tub and get your ass on the toilet before you start gushing. Have some reading material ready, and extra toilet paper. Let the enema do its magic, flushing occasionally to keep from staining the toilet. Once you're past the first ten minutes of letting it go, you can get up from the seat once in awhile for a blood-clot prevention break and to lift the toilet seat to clean up your splashy mess.

You should plan on spending between one to one and a half hours for the entire procedure, once you have the enema in the bag and ready to go.

Enemas as a Regimen

If you have a lot of anal sex, then you should probably give yourself a high colonic every four to eight weeks, depending on how much you eat and how fast your body processes it. Due to the anal sex, your anus may not always get rid of the amount you need it to and the lower intestines can develop a build-up of impacted fecal matter over time. This can become uncomfortable and unhealthy. You can get to where you know your body and you can feel when it's time to "enemize" again. Some go for a quarterly regimen, religiously doing a high coffee colonic every three months. Others, bi-annually. You use your own discretion based on your lifestyle and how much you may need to maintain intestinal fortitude.

To Coffee Enema Or No?

First off: Hot coffee should never be put into your anus! It should be cooled first. If you have high blood pressure or are otherwise avoiding caffeine then you should use decaffeinated coffee for your enemas. Some people have been known to become addicted to coffee enemas, so be moderate in your indulgence.

Chapter 3

Blood

If you're a male and you have a lot of anal sex, you may occasionally notice blood in or on your stool or when you wipe. Your prostate has a protective membrane that tends to break or tear during anal sex, so a little blood as a result of your lifestyle choice is normal. If you start bleeding, then that's not normal and you should seek medical attention and be honest about how you acquired your injury.

Does hairy-ness matter?

Hygiene and maintenance all come together to contribute to the anal sex experience. An anus is already tighter than a vagina, usually, so you want there to be less friction components at play during penetration. Anyone who has ever experienced "hair burn" on his penis can tell you how uncomfortable it can be. And, yes, hair burn is real, does happen, and has been known to cause infection. If you shave it, maintain it. The stubble from not shaving often enough can be just as painful as the grown out hair. Since hair tends to retain odors, shaving down there helps one to control their scent.

Afterwards. After the Sex:

Okay. Many believe that they are all done with everything once they've had their anal sex encounter. But there's still a final process one should always go through for health reasons. After your encounter is completely over with, you should visit the toilet to do the two fingered dig-out to remove any residual lubricant. This is a good health measure. By getting rid of the excess vegetable shortening, you lower the chance of it raising your bad cholesterol levels, a risk you take if you make a habit of skipping this step (leaving it in your anus to get into your bloodstream).

A Side Note About Parachuting:

Do not put pills directly into your anus! If you "parachute", which is a term referring to inserting stimulants into the anus, the preparation step for that is to crush it up and fold it up in a small piece of paper towel, which is then dampened and inserted into the anus.

Some people use muscle relaxers before being on the receiving end of anal sex. Some of the people who do this like to insert the drug into their anus to immediately effect the region they want relaxed and to lessen the effects on the rest of their body. If you parachute prior to anal sex, be sure to remove the parachute before allowing penetration for sex. It can become an aggravating irritant to you and to your partner, or worse.

Water Sports

Drinking Urine

Some people associate it to anal sex, even though neither has anything to do with the other. There's a trick to reducing the risks when indulging in this practice. First off: Drink a lot of fluids before the encounter. The best choice would be water. This should only be done occasionally and only in moderation. Infections have resulted from drinking piss. It comes with risks.

Do not eat feces! Licking anus and sucking anus are okay. But do not eat dukey, ever, not under any circumstances!

Basic Warnings:

Do not put anything into your anus with sharp edges. You could cut your innards!

Do not use glass objects as dildos. You could cut your innards!

Enjoy anal sex in moderation. You could wear-out your innards!

You are now ready to begin.

Vincent Ciofani was born in Detroit, Michigan and was, for the most part, raised there; except for the 4 years his family spent in Alabama when he was a child. Vincent is an accomplished Jazz and Rock guitarist, rapper and lead vocalist who has participated in and produced many Rap songs. Vincent is also a painter and a visual artist and sometimes subcontracts as a videographer for alternative film projects. He currently resides in northern Michigan where he is rumored to be undergoing transformation in a private setting.

Made in United States
Orlando, FL
22 June 2025